Made in United States
North Haven, CT
14 December 2023

45839623R00055